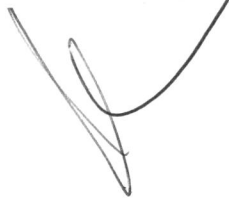

Thirty-Minute Fitness

John Moynihan

Fresh Pond Books
FPB

Thirty-Minute Fitness
Copyright © 2014 by John Moynihan
Fresh Pond Books, Plymouth, Ma.
Library of Congress Control Number: xxxxxxxxxxxxxxx
ISBN: 978-1493605743

This is a work of nonfiction created by John Moynihan.

Published by Fresh Pond Books. Fresh Pond Books publishes contemporary fiction and non-fiction books in a variety of categories and topics of interest. Fresh Pond Books may be purchased for educational, business, or sales and promotional use. For information, please write to Special Marketing, FPB, 64 Linden Place, Brookline, Ma. 02445

Visit www.FreshPondBooks.com

FIRST EDITION

Also by John Moynihan

Canadian Meds
Wampum Nation
The Boomer Survival Guide
The One Hour MBA

To

Sam Moynihan and Jim Sellers

You need to take responsibility for being the healthiest person you can be.

No one else is going to do it for you.

Mehmet Oz, MD

April 2013

Contents

Introduction

Does the world need another exercise book?

Absolutely not.

Then why write this one? And more importantly, why read it once it's written?

This book is a short exercise guide that I believed had to be written for all Americans. By and large, we are a nation of people who don't exercise. This is a mistake. Exercise is the single biggest health benefit that we are in control of in our lives.

We fight like harpies over health care insurance coverage but manage to miss the essential driver of it all—good health.

Many people have significant amounts of energy and enthusiasm and start out on solid exercise programs. Often they are successful in their efforts and look and feel great. They are in good health.

Then something happens. They lose their job and can't afford the health club membership anymore. Or they get sick and stop exercising. Or they twist their ankle. For various reasons, when they get healthy again, they never get back to their exercise routine.

Many times people get bored exercising and just stop.

Circumstances conspire to cause exercise routines to change and ultimately evaporate. Your car breaks down and you can't get to the gym for a week. Your job requires you to travel to Detroit. You go there for two weeks, and it takes you a month to recover and get back into your exercise rhythm. Or Grandma passes away, God rest her soul, and it takes two days to travel to Cleveland and go to the service. While you're there, you make her famous fried chicken recipe for ten people and put on three pounds.

This is all too commonplace.

Exercise is the single most important and controllable health and wellness benefit.

We don't need a prescription from an MD to exercise and get in good health. We don't need to go to a Minute Clinic and wait for a nurse or physician's assistant to tell us to exercise.

No, we just need the willpower to go out and do it. Not a lot, just a little really.

In fact, just thirty minutes a day. Do this four to five times a week, and you will be fit for life.

Just put on the running or jogging shoes and go out and do something. Do almost anything. But do it for thirty minutes a day. And do it for four to five days a week.

That is it.

The ability to get and stay in shape in a time period as short as 30 minutes a day is revolutionary. It's very powerful. This is the time it takes to watch one short show on TV.

Think about that. Who works out in so short a time period? Well, I do for one.

Can it work and be effective? Yes! Absolutely it can. It's like taking an 81 mg aspirin a day.

Simple, yet effective.

Do I exercise regularly? I do. I have been exercising since I was fifteen years old. I was on the crew team in high school and college. With rowing, you are exercising all year long. Running, lifting weights, doing calisthenics—these are the things that oarsmen do. I loved rowing, and that meant I enjoyed exercising. They go together. One of the great benefits, among many, of being on the crew team is that you are always in shape. It comes with the territory.

Rowing ended, but exercising did not. Exercising has always been my true north in many ways.

So this small pocket book is about exercising and how to get and stay in shape. It's not rocket science. It's medical science. Some of it is boring. **But the good news is that it's mostly pretty easy to do. The regimen is**

basic, and you can easily fit it into your life, whatever your circumstances. Trust me on this.

This exercise routine is so simple that you will enjoy doing it and hopefully make it a part of your everyday life. If you follow this guidebook closely, you won't need to spend money on P90X or Zumba or a membership to LA Fitness. You'll already have most of the benefits.

I kept this book short so you can reference it easily and remember all the good info inside.

One last thing. If you haven't exercised for a while and are significantly out of shape, get a medical check-up first before you start. Make sure your MD clears you for moderate exercise. An ounce of prevention is worth a pound of cure here.

Happy exercising!

MINDSET

The Fountain of Youth

There is a real fountain of youth. But it's not in the Florida Everglades, where Ponce de Leon supposedly tramped around in the marsh grass and estuaries, searching for it centuries ago. It's closer. In fact, it's right there in your own basement.

People the world over are looking for the keys to fitness and the fountain of youth. They seek it in the form of juicers, yoga, lavish gyms, holistic medicine, and expensive surgeries. Think pomegranate juice here as an example. The search is endless, and there are mountains of self-help books to get you there.

The good news is that the secret to fitness and good health exists, and I have found it, unlike Ponce de Leon. I found it after fifteen years in the locker room of the Brookline Municipal Swimming Pool.

It's called regular, disciplined exercise. Not exercise that you'd find in an Army or Marine boot camp at five in the morning or that has you running marathons. Just short, regular exercise done consistently.

It's all basic, easy stuff—but it requires discipline and doing it at least four or five times a week.

I was an athlete in both high school and college, so I was no stranger to working out. I also have had three back surgeries (so far!). As I recuperated, I went to municipal and YMCA pools to strengthen my back through swimming. Along the way, I discovered a small tribe of men and women of many different ages, all in good shape.

These people were not ripped, hard-body types—just regular exercisers. The key is that they exercised consistently, and they rarely abandoned their routines. The people I met in the men's locker room were from all across life's spectrum—orthopedic surgeons, college English professors, plumbers, policemen, pharmaceutical reps, artists, and information systems guys.

The only common thread for everyone was regularity and consistency in exercising every week.

That is the key to success.

Lifestyle Choices

You need to incorporate exercise into your lifestyle and daily routine. It's as important as brushing your teeth, eating, or going to work to make money.

Once you include it as a necessity in your daily routine, just like going to work, you will be successful. It will suddenly become easy to maintain your routine.

It's very easy to get out of shape, become stiff, and be lethargic. This can happen when you're thirty years old as easily as when you are fifty. Believe it.

With iPads and smartphones, we spend far too many hours every day being sedentary, trolling the Internet. Not good stuff.

Thirty minutes of exercise has to become part of your mantra, your everyday routine. You can't think about it. You just have to get out there and do it.

Exercise also can become your sweet spot, where you are able to escape and think clearly for a few minutes.

My favorite analogy in terms of staying active and exercising is that of turning an aircraft carrier. These ships are hulking leviathans of the sea. You don't turn an aircraft carrier quickly or easily—it just doesn't respond. Instead, you turn it one degree at a time, and a quarter mile later, it starts to turn, very slowly. Your body is just like that. If you make incremental changes at the helm to move it, it will eventually respond—particularly to exercise.

It happens slowly and over time, but it is powerful.

Exercise Madness

Exercise today has become cult-like for many people. It is all-consuming. People spend hours exercising and are obsessed with their ability to do expensive, time-gobbling, energy-depleting workouts.

There is P90X. There is Zumba. There is CrossFit. There is cardio boxing. There is a world of similar programs. These regimens are usually not cheap. They cost hundreds of dollars to enroll in. Then there are additional costs to maintain them or to get advanced courses as you progress.

Gym memberships are equally expensive. You are often required to pay an initiation fee and then a monthly fee for access to the gym or exercise facility. These fees get costly over time.

These are all great programs and routines. The people who teach them, in addition to being wonderful entrepreneurs looking to make money, are very earnest and passionately believe in their fitness products and message.

Unfortunately, most of these programs are not sustainable over the long term. Very few people can put in the time and energy required month after month to do these routines correctly and consistently.

So, what happens? You cycle. You spend thirty to forty-five days and get in great shape, working out an hour or more a day. You're in the kind of shape you would be in after you finished boot camp in one of the branches of the US military. But, as everyone knows, boot camp doesn't last forever. It is for a definable period and then that's it. It stops.

And that is just what will happen with you or your workouts if you try to do one of the time-consuming routines described above over the long haul. It will stop eventually.

It is all too predictable.

So how do you maintain reasonable fitness with a minimum amount of time and effort?

Read on.

THIRTY-MINUTE FITNESS

Thirty-Minute Fitness

Thirty-Minute Fitness (TMF) is designed to give your body the most substantial exercise benefit in the least amount of time expended.

The goals of the TMF program are simple. One, get in shape so you feel healthy and fit. Two, build a strong core and gain flexibility. Three, maintain a basic level of muscle tone and strength.

That's it! By exercising smart and for no more than thirty minutes a day, you will be in great shape and feel vital.

The essence of Thirty-Minute Fitness is that you have to do some form of exercise most every day to get and stay in shape, but you only have to do a small amount. And that amount is just thirty minutes.

This approach is not a gimmick. It is also not some secret set of exercises that you need a DVD or downloaded app to unlock the mysteries of. It does not require a specialized routine or a trainer to teach you the core elements of the program. It is all just common sense and based on a reasonable and thoughtful approach to exercise.

The TMF program requires focus to do it correctly. It relies on small amounts and levels of exercise and weight training. You are doing fewer exercises with fewer repetitions, but you are doing them correctly and with good form. Focus and form are key.

Thirty-Minute Fitness addresses the need for both strength training and cardiovascular work. They are both critically important elements to your workout routine and fitness goals. You have to do something in both areas daily to stay in shape with Thirty-Minute Fitness.

The best part of Thirty-Minute Fitness is that you are able to vary the mix of both strength and cardio training almost limitlessly with exercises and routines that you are comfortable with. And you are able to—and need to—keep mixing up your routines to, as they say, keep it fresh and real.

Probably the single biggest obstacle to staying in shape is the drudgery of having to exercise every day, doing a routine that is difficult and/or boring. Soon enough, you will find ample reasons or excuses not to workout. And once exercising becomes a burden, you will quickly stop doing it. It is human nature.

Because getting and staying in shape with Thirty Minute-Fitness is not drudgery, you are more inclined and motivated to do your routine every day. Why? Because you never see it as hard. It is actually quite simple—and fun!

The Routine—Two Parts

The secret to success is simple. You have to exercise four to five times a week, doing a basic and consistent routine.

The routine is composed of two parts: One part builds flexibility and strength. One part builds cardiovascular fitness.

Put them together and you have Thirty-Minute Fitness (TMF)—a complete workout that will keep you on course to good health.

Part One—This part is short. Here you do six to ten minutes of core work, exercises, strength training, and weights. You can do calisthenics like jumping jacks or lunges. You can do core exercises to strengthen your center. You can do light weight training with dumbbells or using a bar with weights. Or both. Or all of these things—just mix them up.

Part Two—This part takes twenty to twenty-two minutes. Here you need to go for a walk. Or a run. Or swim for twenty minutes in your local municipal pool. Or ride a spinning bike. You don't have to be super intense here; just do a solid, consistent routine for twenty minutes. You need to mix it up and do different activities every day. Don't do the same thing two or three days in a row. Keep changing the cardio activity you do so that your body gets fit through a variety of things—walking or running, swimming, biking, rowing, whatever.

My favorite aerobic exercises are swimming, biking, and walking. I call it my holy trinity. More on this in the aerobic workout section further on.

The total routine must be short. This is so you can do it daily and so you can fit it into your busy, hectic schedule. The routine also has to be consistently done.

These two elements are the keys to success: short and consistent. The Thirty-Minute Fitness routine needs to have both elements in it to be successful. You need the strength/flexibility part and the cardio part equally.

That is the essence of this book, simply stated. Nothing more. Just do ten minutes of strength training and twenty minutes of cardiovascular training four to five days a week.

Learn and do this consistently for the rest of your life, and you will be fit. You will be in shape, have good health, and feel great.

I guarantee it.

Keep a Journal

You need to keep a journal or log of your fitness activity every day. This is important. It becomes your journal of truth. Use it for everything you do.

By keeping track of your activity every day, you are able to see what it is you have done. Or haven't.

All too frequently we deceive ourselves that we are doing more working out and exercising than we actually are. This is simply human nature. You think that you have exercised four times a week over the past three weeks. Then you look at your log and you see that you did three workouts in one week, four the second week, and only two the third week.

This happens to me all the time. The pool is closed, so I miss a regularly scheduled swim. Or the dog throws up on the living-room rug, and I have to spend twenty minutes cleaning the mess up. I miss my workout, as I've run out of time.

Not good.

By keeping the journal, I am able to track what I have or haven't done each week for exercise. I used to get a small, three-by-five notebook at CVS and go week by week, one week on a page with a short summary of what I did and how long I did it: Swim 22:35 minutes, Walk 25:20 minutes, Exercise Bike 22:15 minutes, etc. I would also add if I had any health issues that I was dealing with that week: cold, flu, stiff neck, sore back, and so on. This approach works well for me, and it's very simple.

You can also keep your log in an Excel spreadsheet on your MacBook Air or smartphone calendar if you prefer. I like to put it on paper and keep it in my gym bag for quick reference. It's old school, but it works.

I have changed a bit over time, and now I use a monthly calendar where I can see an entire month on two pages. This gives me a better perspective visually on my monthly exercising.

This is usually six by nine inches, and I still get it at CVS. Now I have a small square, about one inch in size, to work with and record my daily activity. This is just enough space to write, "Swim 22:15," and the venue. If I am traveling for business and not able to work out or just simply miss a day, I put a zero with a line through it, the null symbol, in that day to indicate that I've missed a day of exercising.

So keep a daily log or journal, and you will have an indelible record of what you've done during the month and eventually the year. This is important for use as a feedback mechanism going forward. It allows you to see how regular you are at exercising and what it is you do most frequently—i.e., where your interests lie.

Look at your results frequently.

Journaling is a critically useful tool, so start your journal the first day you start your Thirty-Minute Fitness program.

KEYS TO SUCCESS

Simple

Keep it simple, stupid. KISS.

In this short acronym, you have the key to success with Thirty-Minute Fitness.

Don't craft routines that are complicated and hard to carry out.

For example, there are hundreds of exercises and calisthenics that you can do as part of your TMF routine. All are beneficial and good.

Just don't try to cram in fifteen of those exercises in each session of eight to ten minutes. It's too much.

Instead, do five or six exercises one day. Then do five or six different exercises the next day.

Always keep your routine simple enough that you can do it without feeling pressured or stressed that you have to do more, more, more.

Doing fewer exercises or weight routines correctly is far better than doing more exercises rushed and with poor form.

You'll also feel more relaxed when doing a simple routine, and that will help maintain your focus and energy. You will feel like you are accomplishing more.

It all translates into a more holistic approach to exercising.

Less really does turn out to be more in the end.

Keep it simple.

Focused

You should always stay focused while you exercise.

This is the corollary to the thought on the previous page: keep your routine simple.

So, on one hand, Thirty-Minute Fitness requires that you do a limited number of calisthenics or exercises or light weight training to start. On the other hand, you've got to have great form and focus on every single repetition that you do during these exercises.

That's because you are usually doing so few repetitions that you have to make every one count. For instance, you may only do seven push-ups in a set. Now, while that's not a large number of push-ups, you have to focus on each one so you execute them with perfect form and approach.

For me, this means no headphones during this first part of the workout.

You can't be thinking about going out to dinner with friends while you are doing your eight to ten minutes of weight training or exercises. You need to be thinking about the exercises and how you move your chest correctly and how your arms should be aligned. You've got to be in the moment.

Less reps, but more focus. That's the trade-off. That's what you have to do to for every exercise.

That way, you get the most out of the minimum.

Focus is the second key to success with your Thirty-Minute Fitness routine.

Don't forget it.

Short

Short and to the point.

This is probably the most important key to doing Thirty-Minute Fitness successfully and consistently.

You need to keep your exercise routine short: the total workout should be no longer than thirty minutes. That's all the time you need from start to finish daily to stay in great shape.

This amount of time spent consistently will put you in the top 10 percent of fit people in the country. Trust me.

There are probably fifty studies that conclude that you need to exercise for forty-five to sixty minutes a day—or walk three miles or swim a mile—for the recommended amount of daily aerobic activity. They are backed up by MDs and PhDs in exercise physiology from the best universities. These studies are all true and proven and scientific.

You need to forget about these studies and do the minimum only. Do the minimum—that's the catchphrase of this key, and it's a critically important one.

The best and most consistent exercisers that I have known through the years are all basically the same:

Get in, get the workout done, get out. Those kind of people.

The doctors, the managers, and the ex-college jocks that I swim with are all twenty- to twenty-five-minute guys, just like me. Specifically, I swim just twenty-two minutes per session. I've been doing it for thirty years, and it's just enough for me.

If I am on my spinning bike, I do a routine that lasts twenty-five minutes.

If I do a walk outside, I walk for no more than twenty-five minutes. The key is to keep it short and simple, doing the minimum only. If the walk takes longer, then cut it down to a length that brings you back to your start within twenty-five minutes—and absolutely no more. If you want to do a long walk on the weekend, that's fine. Just don't do it as part of your daily routine.

I will take twenty to twenty-five minutes of aerobic exercise in some form, daily, or at least frequently, over much longer, less frequent exercise routines. Hands down, it's better.

Regular

Regularity—as in every day—is the final key to exercising.

You need to exercise consistently and repetitively, like going to work or watching TV or doing whatever it is you do. The trick is that you don't have to do big, time-consuming workouts that take forty-five minutes to over an hour to be successful.

Just do light, easy workouts—but ones that you do well and regularly—four to five times a week on an ongoing basis.

Dan Shaughnessy is a well-known Boston sportswriter. He began a program years ago where he would run a mile every day. Not almost every day, but every day. Every single one. He had flights to the West Coast, midnight games, illnesses in his family, time conflicts—basically all the issues that every one of us faces. But he kept on running a mile every day. I don't know if he still does this routine, but it sounds great.

That is exactly the ethic, the mindset that you have to adopt to make an exercise campaign really work. Regularity is key.

Eventually you get sick and miss a week of workouts. Or your job requires you to travel for a week. Or your dog requires an extra twenty-minute walk at night. At that point, you can easily build a mental block about exercising, and you stop doing it. Just like that. It's not a conscious thing, like saying you'll never workout again. It just happens. It creeps in. Life intervenes. And then you're done, and you become another out-of-shape human.

Think I'm kidding? This is what happens to 90 percent of all the exercisers out there without fail.

They blow up, and then they quit. Like clockwork.

But that's not you, because you're mentally prepared and committed to doing short, simple, regular exercise over the long haul.

Consistent

Consistency is key in exercising.

How does this differ from regularity on the previous page? **Regularity relates to keeping a routine during the week. Consistency relates to continuing to work out over a long period**.

If you are able to do your Thirty-Minute Fitness workout consistently over the long haul, you will be successful.

But keeping consistency in your exercise routine is not easy.

In fact, it is probably the hardest part of this program or any program to maintain. This is the area where most people fail.

It's easy to start an exercise program with a tremendous amount of energy and drive. Everybody has the energy necessary to start an exercise regimen. But after you get in shape—say, in thirty or forty-five days—that's where the hard part begins.

Because you have to maintain the energy and discipline needed to continue doing your workouts.

So the key to success in Thirty-Minute Fitness is to always keep the workouts easy enough to do, so that you are always ready and enthusiastic about doing them. Once they become drudgery and/or a chore, you will stop doing them, and your exercise program will quickly end.

This happens to people with the best intentions of staying in shape all the time. They get bored or tired, and they quit. Don't let this happen to you.

Keep doing your routine four to five times a week, week after week, month after month, and you will be successful and feel great.

Flexible

The key to any Thirty-Minute Fitness routine that you craft now is that it be short and flexible.

It must be short enough to fit it into your routine every day, or at least four to five times a week. And it must be flexible enough for you to be able to incorporate different routines when life's bumps come your way.

Three examples come to mind: work travel, injury or pain, and sickness.

Work travel—You need flexibility when you are traveling, particularly for work. You may not be able to do your typical daily routine because you couldn't fit your workout gear into your bag. That's OK. Try borrowing a pair of fitness shoes at the front desk of your hotel, and do something in the hotel gym for fifteen minutes for strength training. Or wear comfortable walking shoes when you travel as your main pair of shoes. Then go for a walk around the city where you are staying before your colleagues get up. Or do it after that big dinner you went to.

Injury—If you've pulled a muscle or strained a ligament or otherwise hurt yourself, you may not be able to do you daily weight training or calisthenics as part of your Thirty-Minute Fitness routine. Not to worry. Go swimming or work out on a spinning bike to make up for it. Work around your injury, and do something that is just as healthy for you but doesn't affect your sore or hurting body part. Don't stop exercising—just workout around your injury.

Being sick—If you're sick with a head cold, don't just scrap your workouts. Sure, it doesn't make sense to go swimming and get all that chlorinated water in your sinuses. And sure, you feel miserable. That's OK. Go for a walk instead. The walk is just as good for you, probably better, and it is something that you can still do when you are sick. Adapt. Work around your sickness.

I call this smart fitness. It entails using your smarts to keep working out and staying fit around all the obstacles and bumps that are put in front of you. You'll need to be very good at juggling exercise all the time to remain on track.

Why? Because, like most people, you'll be confronted with these obstacles every day, and there will always be a reason—a bad reason—not to exercise.

Don't give in, or succumb, to this tendency to skip working out when roadblocks arise.

Fight it, and work around your problems.

Stop—Don't Do More!

Resist the temptation—don't do more.

This is one of the key concepts of Thirty-Minute Fitness. Do not forget it.

The typical exercise training routine is founded on the more-is-better approach.

More. More. More. Always do better. Always push to do more.

If you can do ten push-ups, then eventually you can do eleven. And then twelve. And then on up to fifteen. You know, keep *pushing* yourself. Soon fifteen push-ups is your new baseline. You will then always need to do fifteen push-ups, then twenty. Always.

The theory is that doing more is good for you and that you'll get stronger along the way.

I can pretty much tell you that if you go on this kind of exercise routine, you are very likely to fail over time, as the routine quickly becomes overbearing and you burn out. Soon you don't want to do any exercise at all—that is, you don't go back to doing fewer repetitions. You just stop altogether because you get frustrated and worn out.

This happens to most people almost all the time.

Let me say it again: This happens to almost everybody all the time!

If you build up to bigger workouts with more repetitions or longer times, you'll build the proverbial battleship. A World War II era battleship had a small keel and waterline and a big, heavy superstructure. When you build that superstructure up high enough, the ship has a tendency to topple over in rough weather, because it's top-heavy with extraneous stuff. That's you with your exercise routine. You'll topple over in the first storm that hits your life, and you'll immediately stop exercising.

Don't let this happen. Keep it simple. Do your allotted routine, whatever you decide, but don't do more. Just stop and enjoy the extra time you have.

Keep your sets short, simple, and fixed.

Marginal Benefits

Most Americans go for supersizing everything, especially food, drink, and the homes they live in.

This also extends to their workouts. Going big is considered good. As in, go big or go home.

Surprisingly, in the exercise world, bigger is often *not* better.

A variety of studies have shown that people get 75 to 80 percent of the full benefit of a workout in a routine that lasts about twenty to twenty-five minutes. That's all you need! In fact, a lot of exercise scientists add that you can break your workout up during the day and do ten minutes here and ten minutes there.

To get the extra benefit of the final 25 percent of a workout, a person may have to put in an additional thirty to forty-five minutes. So the extra time you spend in a longer workout is wildly disproportional to the marginal benefit you receive.

It is simply not efficient.

Why not do the minimum and get 80 percent of the benefit you need? Energy is precious, and expending too much for so little return is not logical.

Now, no doctor or personal exercise trainer is likely to support a routine that is this short. Most recommend forty-five to sixty minutes of vigorous activity. Less is not enough.

Fuhgeddaboudit!

This is a fitness regimen that is geared to give you the maximum benefit for the least amount of work. This isn't a Gold's Gym workout routine or a training program for a marathon.

You only need to be in reasonably good shape to be successful in life.

And Thirty-Minute Fitness gets you there.

Mix It Up: Cross-Train

So there you have it—jogging, biking, walking, or swimming. Do those four exercises twenty to twenty-five minutes a day, and you've got it nailed for the rest of your life. Throw in six to ten minutes of exercises or light weight training on top of that, and you've got a stellar, all-star workout routine that can all be done in thirty minutes. That's right, thirty minutes.

That's Thirty-Minute Fitness in a nutshell.

The last key to success in doing this routine effectively is to cross-train.

This is a sophisticated way of saying, "Mix it up."

You need to alternate the entire program constantly—the exercises, the calisthenics, the light weight training, and the aerobic activity. Constantly and continually change things.

Doing something most days is ideal, but just don't do the same thing day in and out.

Like swimming? Don't swim seven days a week, because before you know it, you'll have a sore elbow or a stiff shoulder and hate swimming.

Like running? Don't do it five days in a row, because you'll end up with a hot knee, and it will become stiff and sore, and you won't want to run again—ever.

Like biking? If you ride your bike frequently and are using drop-down handlebars, there's a fairly good chance that you'll irritate your neck from riding in a hunched over position.

All these problems are fairly typical for people who exercise in the same way frequently and generally can be easily fixed.

Just be sure that you cross-train, that you alternate workouts so you use different muscle groups every day. Use the exercise bike one day, go swimming the next day, and run or walk for twenty to twenty-five minutes the third day.

That is all the sophisticated exercise planning that you need to do. Nothing more than that.

THE GYM

Efficiency

Why get a home gym?

Why spend the money and the time to outfit one? The answer, in a word, is simple: efficiency.

When you have a gym in your spare room or basement, you are right off the top able to save fifteen to twenty minutes a day when working out.

That's because you don't have to drive or walk to a gym where you have to check in, change, and then jockey for exercise space in a big room with everybody else.

The absolute key to Thirty-Minute Fitness and doing the program successfully is to have it be as frictionless as possible.

By frictionless, I mean the ability to make your program easy and effortless. Of making it simple and fun and something that you want to do daily. That's frictionless.

By far, the task that causes the most friction for most people is the effort that you have to expend to get to the gym to exercise in the first place.

By making a gym right in your home or apartment, you are able to do your Thirty-Minute Fitness routine immediately.

And doing it immediately is the single way that will make you successful in doing it over and over, for the long haul. If it is not easy and accessible, over time you will tend to skip your workouts. That is fatal to your fitness success.

Remember: efficiency matters.

Gym Basics

Do you need a real gym, a separate space to work out in to do Thirty-Minute Fitness every day?

No! Not at all.

Then why bother? Space is hard enough to find in our apartments and houses for essential things like closets and bedrooms, so a gym may seem frivolous.

My point is that a "gym" should be your exercise room in the metaphorical sense, a place where you go each day to do your exercises.

It can be in your bedroom, in your basement, in your living room, or in your garage.

Just have a quiet spot where you can exercise without distraction, stretch fully, and not knock things off the wall or hit your arms or head on the ceiling.

If you are pressed for space, your bedroom is fine. Just keep your key pieces of exercise equipment under your bed and easy to get at every day.

What should you have in your gym for exercise equipment if you do have the extra room and want to set up a separate place to exercise?

This is the easy part, because it probably consists of six to eight items that don't cost more than $150 to outfit yourself for what you need to exercise successfully.

I think one or two sets of dumbbells is necessary—one set of five-pound dumbbells and one set of ten-pound dumbbells. You want to have one lighter set to use to loosen up with and one heavier set for basic muscle resistance when you do weight-training exercises.

Also, get two rubber resistance bands. One should be relatively easy to pull and the other should be moderately harder. A lot of professional athletes use resistance bands now, and they are great. More on resistance bands in a few pages.

I also suggest a set of handgrips to develop hand and forearm strength. You may also want a set of push-up stands. They cost twenty dollars and allow you to do push-ups correctly. Total outlay here is less than $150, for sure.

That's it for the absolute basics, the minimum that you need for your gym. One of the many beauties and simplicities of your own home gym is that you can build and customize it over time. Add a small piece of exercise equipment every six months or so. But make sure you actually use all the items you have. If you don't use something, get rid of it, so that you only have equipment that is essential and functional for your fitness.

My Gym

I have a home gym in my basement.

It's a small, converted room that the previous owner's kids used during high school for hanging out.

If you're curious, I'll tell you what I have in my own gym so you'll know for comparison. It's a little more than your basic gym, but not by much. I've got the following:

- A full set of dumbbells in pairs ranging from three to twenty pounds. This is so I can start light and go heavier during my workout. But I rarely use the twenty-pound dumbbells. They're there for show only.
- Two different exercise bands for resistance training. One is very light and easy to pull. The second has more resistance.
- A simple exercise bench to do leg lifts to build my core and for bench pressing.

- A set of push-up stands to do push-ups correctly. Push-ups are great exercises, but you've got to do them right to get any benefit.
- Two sets of handgrips, one easy and one hard. This is for developing hand and forearm strength.
- Framed posters of Michael Jordan, Muhammad Ali, Tiger Woods, and Tom Brady on the wall for motivation and inspiration.

Equipment:

I also have two pieces of large exercise equipment:

- A good-quality spinning bike that I got at a fitness store for cross-training.
- A good treadmill that I use for walking or running indoors when the weather outside is bad.

That's it! That is pretty much my entire gym that I have been using for over twenty years for exercising. I used to have a big bench press with weights, but I found it cumbersome, so I got rid of it. I also bought other pieces of expensive equipment over time. But if I didn't use them, I quickly sold or gave them away because space is precious in my gym.

So you can see that you don't need a lot to stay in shape. Having a basic gym in place in your home makes it easy to access and do your daily routine. It gives you an efficiency edge and less of a reason not to exercise.

Remember, if it's not easy to exercise, you won't do it. Bet on it.

Resistance Bands

There is a new exercise regimen today done with rubber resistance bands, and it works great.

Resistance bands are great for muscle toning and basic fitness. So go to Dick's or The Sports Authority and buy several bands of different resistance levels, and incorporate them into your exercise routine.

A variety of professional athletes use rubber bands for resistance training, particularly NFL skill players who are highly conditioned athletes.

I use them daily for simple, strengthening exercises for my arms and shoulders. I pull against them in various positions for eight to ten repetitions and quickly do four or five exercises to build flexibility in my neck, arms, and shoulders. They are great for simple resistance training.

My neck and shoulders are frequently problem areas, with pain and stiffness. It's not surprising, since I sit at a desk all day, working at two computer screens. **Resistance**

bands are excellent for keeping your neck and shoulders loose, strong, and flexible.

Put them into your Thirty-Minute Fitness routine, and you'll get the same results.

CORE WORK

Core Importance

Maintaining a strong core is critically important to your fitness. The core is your center and includes your abdominal and back muscles, obliques, and hip flexors. By doing exercises that work these muscle groups and other related ones, you will build a protective sheath around yourself.

Having a strong core is essential to having good posture and a strong, flexible back. I know, because I am a back sufferer. After three surgeries, I really understand the need to have a strong core for back support. Your abdominal muscles are the most obvious and easiest ones to work on here. But your hip flexors and gluteus muscles are important too.

With a solid core, you will ensure that you will be fit for everyday living, working out, participating in athletics, and just feeling good. It will help you sitting down at a desk, lifting objects, walking, and maintaining good posture.

The core controls all your body movements from the center out, so you can't do too much to strengthen and maintain it.

Sit-Ups

Doing sit-ups is a basic and obvious choice to develop core strength.

But be sure to do bent-leg sit-ups so that you don't put stress and strain on your lower back. Lie down on the floor face up, and bend your knees at a forty-five-degree angle, with your feet flat on the floor.

Lock your hands behind your head and come up from this lying down position, slowly and as far as you can. It will only be about eight to ten inches that you'll be able to lift your head and back off the floor. That's enough.

What you are doing is essentially a crunch that is working your abdominal muscles very effectively.

Do one or two sets of seven to ten repetitions here. That's enough. Maintain good form.

Bicycles

This is a great variation of a sit-up that works a variety of muscles in your core.

Lie on the floor face up with your arms over your chest.

Come up into a crunch position. Raise your legs and simulate a bicycle movement, as though you are pedaling an imaginary bike.

Pedal slowly to really work your abdominal core.

Do this for five to ten seconds. Your abs should be tired. This is a tough exercise to do correctly.

Watch your form, go slowly, and really feel the effect on your abdominal muscles.

Do one or two sets for ten seconds each of this exercise for the best effect for building your abdominals.

Leg Lifts

This is another good abdominal and core exercise.

Again, lie flat on your back on the floor.

Keep your hands by your side, and out a little to act as stabilizers for your legs.

Raise your legs up to a forty-five-degree angle and do short scissor kicks, moving your legs up and down in about a twelve- to eighteen-inch movement. Do ten of these kicks.

Bring your legs down to the floor, rest, and then lift and repeat for ten kicks.

To work different parts of your abdominal muscles, change your leg position, so that you kick higher or lower each successive time.

As an alternative, also move your legs sideways in a scissor motion, doing the classic scissor kick. This is a great exercise to work your oblique muscles and is very complimentary to doing leg lifts.

Do two or three sets per workout.

If you can't do sit-ups, this is a great substitute.

Planks

This is a great strengthening exercise for your core. So incorporate it into your routine.

Lie on the floor facedown.

Raise yourself up on your forearms and your toes—with just those touching the floor—like you are starting a push-up.

You have now assumed the position and the look of a plank—a board-like pose where your core and back is ramrod straight and stiff.

Hold this position for five to ten seconds, relax, then hold it again.

For variation, you can raise one leg off the ground five to eight inches and hold it there for three seconds for extra difficulty and strengthening. Raise each leg five times.

That's it for core strengthening exercises. You can always go to the web and get about five to ten additional core exercises and workout tips if you are interested in building up your abdominal and related muscle groups more fully as part of your Thirty-Minute Fitness routine.

FIRST PART: EXERCISES

Calisthenics

Exercises and light weight training are the two front-end activities that you need to do every day as part of Thirty-Minute Fitness. Exercises are the easiest, as they usually require next to nothing in terms of advanced training, talent, or equipment.

The most basic exercises are called calisthenics, and they are back in vogue in many fitness plans. They should definitely be part of your routine.

Calisthenics come from the ancient Greeks and were originally related to Greco-Roman wrestling. The Spartans did calisthenics before battles. Over time, these became known as light exercises designed to promote general fitness and develop muscle tone. They are usually done without any equipment.

Calisthenics are old-school exercises, a throwback to the World War II era training at boot camps to get GIs in shape. They are basic and powerful, and no

equipment is required—just you and your body weight for resistance.

I think calisthenics are an excellent fit for any Thirty-Minute Fitness routine.

My favorites are jumping jacks, lunges, push-ups, sit-ups, leg lifts, crunches, squats, and flutter kicks. There are many variations on these basic exercises.

Calisthenics are a holistic approach to exercise. It is just you and your body. My goal when doing them is to build a basic level of strength, conditioning, and muscle tone.

A variety of calisthenics are discussed in this section, along with a sample routine and some key thoughts on doing the exercises.

Exercise Routine

The following are the basic exercises that I do as part of my Thirty-Minute Fitness training on most days. Alternate doing these exercises with the light weight training discussed in the next section.

Do different exercises to cross-train, avoid injuries, and maintain some variety in your workout. Doing the same ones over and over will lead to boredom, and you'll quit.

Here are the exercises:

- **Jumping jacks**—This is the basic high school exercise. They're great! Do about ten to fifteen repetitions (or reps) for flexibility.
- **Lunges**—Basically, put one leg out in front and then lower yourself slowly, parallel to the ground. This is great for muscle stretching and flexibility. You may have to put your hand on a wall or hold a chair if your balance is bad.

- **Full or half push-ups**—Do two sets of five to ten reps.
- **Arm pulls** with rubber resistance bands—Tie a resistance band on a door knob or a column in your basement, and use it for resistance training for your arms, neck, and shoulders. Create two to three exercises here.
- **Leg lifts off floor**—Lie on the floor or on an exercise bench and lift your legs, scissor-like, about twelve inches off the floor to work your abdominal muscles. You can do these in a variety of positions to isolate various parts of your stomach and core. This is an excellent exercise and one of my favorites.

For all of these exercises, I suggest you do no more than eight to ten repetitions. Do one set of these five exercises, possibly two sets maximum, and that's enough for your daily TMF routine.

Here again, experiment with a wide variety of exercises until you find five or six that are the best for you in terms of conditioning, strength training, and enjoyment.

Circuit Training

Try to do your exercises in a routine that is quick and focused.

So, start with ten push-ups. After you finish, immediately go on to doing ten to fifteen jumping jacks. Then go directly into doing lunges.

Go nonstop from one exercise to the next until you finish your entire routine in this manner.

You don't necessarily need to be fast doing each exercise, just be methodical. Do one exercise correctly and with good form, then go on to the next and then the next without stopping between exercises.

You will start to get winded quickly if you do your exercises without stopping, so you start to get some cardiovascular benefit as well from doing them in a continuous circuit.

Basically, you are doing a circuit of five to seven exercises, without stopping between exercises, while doing each with good form and technique. (You'll see more on good form on the next page, because it's critical to your success here.)

The advantage of circuit training is that it allows you to do five to seven exercises quickly and efficiently.

If you stop between exercises, you waste time, and you won't be able to do as many different exercises before you move on to the aerobic portion of your Thirty-Minute Fitness workout.

Both parts are important, and the circuit training allows you to do your exercise routine quickly.

Form Counts Most

Always use good form.

Give me five absolutely perfect push-ups rather than ten sloppy ones. That's the true secret to exercising success.

This may seem like a small point, but it's not. Form counts the most when exercising—the absolute most. You have to pay strict attention to form for every exercise you do or weight you lift.

Because you're doing fewer repetitions with Thirty-Minute Fitness, you have to pay close attention to your form for each rep to get maximum benefit from the fewer that you do. You'll do fewer reps, but excellent ones.

Repetitions don't count. You don't get credit for doing twenty sloppy crunches. You get a demerit instead.

It is far better to do smaller sets of different exercises, maybe four or five different ones, but do each set impeccably well. How small? Sets of five to seven repetitions of lunges, curls, half push-ups, and jumping jacks are all fine, in my opinion.

You have to stay focused on form and posture for each and every repetition. Do each repetition slowly, and concentrate on your form. That's the key to working your muscles effectively. If you focus on each push-up and get the maximum benefit from each repetition, then you don't need to do fifteen repetitions.

Just squeeze each rep out perfectly.

By keeping the sets small and varied, you also avoid injury.

There's another benefit to the idea of small, focused sets of repetitions, and it's psychological. If you keep your sets small, you'll always want to do them, even on the days when working out is the last thing you want to do.

Again, that's the key to Thirty-Minute Fitness. You need to keep everything simple, focused, and easy to do.

On the following pages are some of my favorite exercises that I do and that you can also do as part of your TMF routine.

Push-Ups

If I had to pick only one exercise to do, push-ups would be the choice.

When done right, they are a great overall exercise for the body, especially for your chest, shoulders, and back.

Full push-ups—Lie on the floor facedown. Put your palms on the floor at the position of your shoulders. Raise your body up in a straight line, keeping your back, legs, and shoulders rigid. Your arms are doing all the work.

Do two sets of five to ten push-ups per set, depending on how strong and fit you are. You can start small here, doing two to three reps and then gradually building up. It's better to do fewer push-ups, but do each one with good form.

Half push-ups—One trick you can use is to do half push-ups, or push-ups from the kneeling position. This is much less stressful on your shoulders and chest and a lot easier. I only do half push-ups as part of my Thirty-Minute Fitness routine because they're easier and I can isolate my chest and shoulders and do seven to ten great technique push-ups every time.

The key is that I watch my form closely, and I keep each one crisp so that every repetition counts. I keep the repetition count low so that I can do each push-up strongly and smoothly.

One other trick I have is to use a set of push-up stands when doing this exercise. You can get them at The Sports Authority or Dick's, and they isolate your chest and arms so that you are forced to use good form when doing this exercise. They are great! They cost about twenty dollars and will last a lifetime.

Flutter Kick

This is a great exercise for your abdominal muscles.

I usually do two sets of flutter kicks, fifteen reps in each set.

Lie flat on your back and put your hands under your butt for stability.

Now raise your feet twelve inches off the floor and kick them as a swimmer would do during a freestyle event.

You can feel the tension in your abs as you kick. Keep your kicks short and tight, moving your legs no more that twelve to fifteen inches as you kick.

You can do a variation of this kick by raising your torso up and kicking your feet at a higher angle, say forty-five degrees from the floor.

Do two or three sets with your legs at a different angle each time so that you work your abdominal muscles slightly differently for each set.

This is a great and easy exercise to build abdominal or core strength.

Jumping Jacks

This is another great, old-school exercise.

Jumping jacks are not particularly hard to do. In fact, they are easy if you just keep your range of motion small and tight.

Jump to a position where your legs are spread out and your hands almost touch above your head.

Then retract your feet and bring your arms back to a position at your side.

Repeat for a set of ten to fifteen.

Do two sets.

If you want to make the exercise easy, only spread your legs about twenty-four inches as you jump and have your arms bent at your elbows as you raise them above your head.

To make it harder, just spread your legs out farther as you jump, and keep your arms straight as you move them in a wider arc above your head.

Deep Knee Bends

This is a good exercise for your legs and back, your hamstrings, quadriceps, and calves.

Stand up, hands by your sides.

Slowly squat down, moving your arms outward to stabilize yourself as you drop down.

Stop at the point where your thighs are parallel to the floor, and hold that positions for two seconds.

Your arms should be directly and fully out in front of you.

Slowly rise up, bringing your arms back down to your sides.

Go lower and deeper on each successive knee bend until you are down at a full squat position, again with your arms out in front of you.

Do two sets of five to seven deep knee bends per set for maximum effect.

Arm Pulls

This is an exercise that you do with rubber resistance bands.

Have the bands attached to a wall or a pole that is strong and solid.

Stand away from the wall with the band just firmed up. Hold the handle with your wrist facing upward.

Your feet should be flat and parallel to your shoulders.

Bring your arm backward in a straight motion as you stretch the band.

Pull back about twenty-four inches for resistance. Make sure that you are using a band that has only medium resistance, as you want to be able to move your arm backward with little effort.

Do ten to fifteen repetitions for each arm.

This is a great exercise to build arm and shoulder strength. The key component here is to use a light resistance band that is not too hard to pull.

Squat Thrusts

Start from a standing position.

Here you'll perform a motion where you first squat down and have your hands touch the floor.

Then kick your legs out so that you are basically in the position of being ready to do a push-up.

But you don't do a push-up.

You bring your legs back in, then stand up again to a full standing position.

Then repeat the entire movement.

Squat—kick out—come back in—stand up.

That's the squat thrust. It can be hard to do.

Like every exercise, it's better to do fewer repetitions while keeping good form for each one.

Do one set of five to ten repetitions.

FIRST PART: WEIGHT TRAINING

Strength

You should lift weights at least two to three times a week as part of your Thirty Minute Fitness program, as muscle strength is a foundation of overall fitness. It strengthens your core, helps your flexibility, and increases your ability to do endurance work as well.

I like to lift light weights every day as part of my own TMF routine. I do only a few weight training exercises, but I do them regularly. I particularly focus on my arms, shoulders, and neck, as I have a tendency to slouch and have occasional neck problems. Strong shoulder and neck muscles help me maintain good posture and keep me pain-free.

The weights you lift as part of Thirty-Minute Fitness should be light weights.

Light weights are usually dumbbells that vary in weight from five pounds to fifteen pounds. My experience is that weights over fifteen pounds are too heavy for most people and are a little cumbersome.

Get four pairs of dumbbells that are five, ten, twelve, and fifteen pounds. These are perfect.

The ones that you will likely use the most are the ten-pound dumbbells. They are great for a variety of exercises, because they build strength, yet they are easy to handle.

Remember here that you are only trying to get into general fitness shape. Getting and staying strong is part of that goal, but building bulk is not.

By lifting light weights, you'll get strong and develop body and muscle tone. You will build good arm and leg strength along the way as well. But because you are not lifting heavy weights, you will not build dense muscle.

It's the difference between building bulk and building firmness.

Firmness is what you want for the long haul to stay in shape. Firmness will support you in everyday living and allow you to participate in a wide variety of sports and activities.

Sample Weight Routine

Lifting light weights is important to maintaining strength and flexibility.

Light is good, as it allows you to focus on perfect form and do each exercise correctly. I suggest you do these exercises in sets of five to seven repetitions. That's all you need, as you're just toning and building basic muscle strength.

Before you start weight lifting, you may want to do a session or two with a personal trainer who is versed in light weight training and can show you good form and technique. You don't need to spend a lot of money or sign up for fifteen sessions. In just one or two sessions, you'll learn the basics.

Remember, there are literally hundreds of similar exercises you can do with light dumbbells or bar weights or even kettle bells which are now in vogue. These exercises are just a start. Find some you like from the web, and incorporate them into your TMF program. Experiment, get creative, and make up a short, focused routine.

Here is a sample of the first part weight training work I do as part of my TMF routine.

- **Curls**—Just back up against a wall and lift the dumbbells up with your elbow against the wall to isolate a good, clean motion.
- **Side dumbbell lift**—Stand relaxed with a dumbbell in each hand, looking straight ahead. Raise the weight up from your side until it is straight out from your body, parallel to the floor. Then lower it. Do the left side and then the right.
- **Military dumbbell press**—Stand straight with a dumbbell in each arm at chest height. Now press both dumbbells up over your head and then return. Basically, this is a standing press.
- **Pectoral front dumbbell lift**—Start out just like the side dumbbell lift, but raise the weight in front of you, bringing it up in front of your chest parallel to the floor, working your chest muscles. Then let the weight back down.
- **Behind-the-head pullover**—Stand straight with one dumbbell behind your head, held with both hands. Now slowly raise it up behind your head until your arms are fully extended and the

dumbbell is directly over your head. Then slowly let it back down.

- **Bench press with dumbbells**—Lie on an exercise bench and do the basic bench press movement using two light dumbbells for resistance.

Experiment and find six to seven exercises that you like to help you build strength and muscle tone. Rotate new exercises in and familiar ones out to keep your routine fresh and varied.

On the next several pages, I have some additional tips on my exercise routine above.

Curls

This is a weight training exercise that I regularly keep in my routine.

I like curls as they build basic arm, forearm, and bicep strength very easily.

I usually isolate my biceps by standing up against a wall or a doorway and lift a single dumbbell up from a straight arm position to a full curl, almost touching my bicep.

I use a fifteen-pound dumbbell and do five repetitions in a set.

And I do two sets for each arm. No more.

Because I do curls almost every day, I keep the repetition count low. If I don't, I find that my elbows start to hurt.

I focus on each curl and make every repetition precise.

Pectoral Dumbbell Lift

This is an exercise that I do to build my chest. It develops the pectoral muscles as well as the arms and the shoulders.

I use ten-pound dumbbells for this exercise.

I begin with both dumbbells in front of me, at my thighs, with my arms hanging down.

I then raise one dumbbell up, keeping my arm straight, so that the weight comes up and the movement stops with the weight directly in front of me, parallel to the floor, at chest level. I then lower it down the same way.

I do five repetitions for each arm for one set. Left arm, then right arm. I do two sets.

Again, using light weights is ideal for doing this basic exercise.

Pullovers

This is a great exercise for the upper back, neck, and arms.

I use a twelve-pound dumbbell for this exercise.

I stand straight with my feet shoulder width apart.

I hold the dumbbell by the end and position it behind my head at the level of my neck.

I then bring the dumbbell up in an arc behind my head and end the motion with the weight directly over my head.

I lower the dumbbell basically in a reverse motion and end with the weight again behind my head.

I do one set of twelve repetitions for this exercise.

This exercise strengthens the neck muscles and provides good support for the head.

Bench Press with Dumbbells

Doing a bench press with dumbbells is arguably harder than doing a bench press with weights on a bar. That's because you have to control each arm separately, and it's harder to have good form while you are pressing both weights independently.

I start by lying flat on an exercise bench with my feet off the floor on the bench and my legs at a forty-five-degree angle. I use fifteen-pound dumbbells to do bench presses, raising them off the ground and over my chest to start. I lower the dumbbells fully to my chest and then slowly raise them back up to a straight-arm position over my head.

I do two sets of seven repetitions.

I am careful to use good technique for each and every repetition I do. Again, lighter weights with good technique equal better results.

This exercise is good for the chest and pectoral muscles, arms, and shoulders.

Military Dumbbell Press

This exercise is the basic press, but it is done standing up rather than lying down.

I use two ten-pound dumbbells here.

With my feet shoulder-width apart, I raise the dumbbells to chest height. Then I press them up and over my head until my arms are fully extended and locked over my head. I then let the weight down to chest level again to end the repetition.

I do one set of 10 reps.

This exercise is good for your spine, back, shoulders, and arms. You must have a straight back to do the exercise correctly.

Use lighter weights here to focus on your form and not stress your back or spine.

Side Dumbbell Lifts

This exercise is similar to the pectoral dumbbell lift.

But here you raise the dumbbells out sideways from your body until your arms are outstretched and are parallel to the floor, and then lower them back down to the starting position. That is one repetition. Do one arm at a time.

Start this exercise with your legs spread apart at shoulder width. Hold the dumbbells down on the left and right side of your body.

With the pectoral lift, you lift the weights up in front of you. With the side lift, you lift the weights up and out from your side. I use ten-pound dumbbells to be able to concentrate on my form throughout this exercise.

This is a great exercise for building abdominal strength and strength in your arms and shoulders.

I use 10-pound dumbbells here to be able to concentrate on my form throughout this exercise.

That's it for tips for my favorite weight-training exercises. Develop your own routine that is easy and has similar characteristics.

SECOND PART: AEROBIC WORKOUTS

Thirty-Minute Fitness—Aerobic Exercise

First do your core work, calisthenics, or weight training. The variety and possibilities here are endless, as you've seen in the earlier sections of this book. This first part should take you no more than ten minutes.

For the next twenty minutes in the second part, you need to participate in a calorie-burning, aerobic-type fitness activity. This is the cardiovascular part. You've got to do something that is active and gets your heart rate elevated.

A wide range of activities qualify here.

They include all the obvious ones—biking, spinning, running, jogging, walking, swimming, basketball, tennis, and hiking.

They can also include walking your dog if it's brisk enough and he or she doesn't stop every five minutes to pee at a tree.

The key here is to do something constant and repetitive that uses up energy and makes you fit.

The absolutely easiest thing to do is leave your house and walk or jog in your neighborhood for twenty minutes.

Start immediately once you get outside, and begin and end right back in front of your house. Minimize any warm-up or cooldown, because that will add time and take you well beyond your thirty minutes.

Try to avoid doing this and using additional time. Why?

Because keeping your total workout to thirty minutes is the real magic of Thirty-Minute Fitness.

It really means what it says—thirty minutes.

The Exercise Benefit

Here's some good news.

If you are doing the first part exercises and weight training that I describe in the earlier sections quickly, you are already likely getting some aerobic benefit from them.

The key is to do them in a circuit-training mode. Again, that means you do your exercises or calisthenics nonstop.

So start with jumping jacks. Then progress immediately to deep knee bends. After you finish those, get on the floor and do sit-ups or flutter kicks to strengthen your core and abdominal muscles. Don't rest between exercises. Then do five to ten push-ups. Complete your routine nonstop.

The key is to do sets with a small number of repetitions, typically seven to ten. That small number of reps allows you to focus on your technique, which is absolutely important, while still getting the benefit of the exercise.

If you are doing weights on a particular day, do your side dumbbell lift, then your military press, then your behind-the-head pullovers quickly and in successive sets.

The key is not to stop.

By doing your first part work in this way, you will have already jump-started your aerobic workout.

Your heart rate will be slightly elevated, and you will be breathing with an aerobic capacity.

This is exactly the way you want to move into the second part of Thirty-Minute Fitness, the aerobic part.

My Holy Trinity

In New Orleans, they have a mixture of vegetables and seasoning that they call the holy trinity. It's green bell peppers, garlic, and celery. Local cooks in New Orleans add these ingredients to almost everything.

The same is true for aerobic work. The holy trinity of cardio activity in my case is lap swimming, biking, and walking or jogging. No handball, basketball, tennis, or running for me. I alternate these three activities routinely and do no more than a twenty-two-minute daily workout doing one of these three.

Swim, walk, bike. Repeat.

These are among the best activities for getting in shape and staying in shape.

Why? They vary the focus on different muscle groups, they're basic, and they're easy to do. Equally important, all three exercises are low impact. Low impact means that you can do these exercises regularly and not hurt yourself by doing them, generally speaking.

These are my favorites, but they may not be yours.

You may prefer running, handball, using a rowing or elliptical machine, tennis, hiking, or using a treadmill. These are all viable alternatives, and just as good or better for building aerobic fitness.

I tend toward routines that are not jarring, good for my back, and relatively easy to do. Notice I don't run. I walk briskly. I probably could jog or run, but for the impact that it would put on my body, I just don't see the benefit. With Thirty-Minute Fitness, I try to do activities that are supportive of my particular body type and known weaknesses, so that I don't aggravate them.

One of the major benefits of Thirty-Minute Fitness is that the workouts are designed to be short—and for a reason. The reason is that short workouts are easier to do and don't tax or stress the body as much. This is an important concept. If you don't work out as much, you don't put heavy stress on your elbows, joints, knees, and hips.

Over time, all exercisers develop some long-term physical challenges: a bad back, a rotator cuff issue, a weak knee or elbow, a painful hip, or a cervical problem. It just happens when working out regularly over a long period.

With TMF, the goal is to keep the workouts light and less stressful.

You'll never do a five-mile run with TMF. Why? It's too long! And more importantly, you don't need it to get fit and stay in basic shape.

For most people who work, have kids, or have other responsibilities in life, my exercises are the easiest and most logical ones to quickly and seamlessly integrate into your lifestyle.

Which is what Thirty-Minute Fitness is all about.

Craft your own holy trinity of activities that you can do in your Thirty-Minute Fitness routine on a regular basis. And then start doing them.

Remember: the aerobic activities that you choose need to be enjoyable and also be ones that you can do quickly and without a lot of preparation or wasted time.

Enjoyment and efficiency are the keys to maintaining your exercise program. They are related.

On the following pages, I riff a bit more about my holy trinity of aerobic exercises.

Swimming

Swimming is possibly the best exercise in the world.

All you need is a bathing suit and a pair of goggles.

You are able to work out with minimal stress and impact on your body.

You can go fast or slow, and can easily isolate different muscles groups with various strokes.

The best part of swimming is that you can have a variety of physical problems and still swim regularly. That's because swimming is very low impact—the water supports your weight. You're floating.

Swimming is also superb for your arms and shoulders.

And if you use a kickboard, you can isolate your abdominal muscles with the flutter kick and strengthen and build your core.

You can get in good shape fast with swimming, because it works many muscle groups simultaneously with minimum body impact.

Most people hate swimming.

Or at least it's not at the top of their fun-activities-to-do list.

Why do they hate swimming?

Well, they're in the water. And it's not always warm. Their head is in the water, and it's often uncomfortable. More significantly, they also have to go to a pool to swim, so logistics play a big role.

These are all small inconveniences, but they add up and can cause enough friction for most people to decide quickly that swimming is not for them.

Some people also just don't like swimming or are not good at it. And that's fine. Just find another activity to substitute here.

It's my number-one aerobic activity in my Thirty-Minute Fitness routine. If I could do only one aerobic exercise, I would swim.

Biking

Biking is another of my personal favorite Thirty-Minute Fitness aerobic activities.

I use a stationary spinning bike for this exercise.

You can get one at BJ's for about $350.

I have one in my basement gym and exercise for twenty-two to twenty-five minutes on it when I do my bike workout. I am usually reading a book while I pedal or watching news or sports on a wall-mounted flat-screen TV.

I also have an old Raleigh cross-training bike that I ride outside all the time in my neighborhood when I do local errands.

It's great to beat traffic, get around town, and stay in shape at the same time.

Biking is a great aerobic exercise because it's another low-impact activity. There's little stress.

There's no pounding (like running), and it is more of a continuous and fluid movement.

Biking works your back, legs, arms, and core very effectively.

Walking

Walking is the third leg of my holy trinity. For most people, walking will be their primary aerobic exercise.

It is possibly the best exercise in the world.

You can do it anywhere.

You only need a pair of running or walking shoes. You can do it in any weather, and you can start immediately once you're out the door.

You don't need a lot of warm-up or cooldown for this activity either. Just get outside and walk.

Walking is also great because you can go slow, fast, or in between. You choose.

Brisk walking is an excellent overall aerobic activity. It works your arms and legs, your back, and your hips.

It strengthens your abdominal muscles as well, so it's great for your core. Walking works many muscle groups very effectively, in a low stress manner.

That's what makes walking so good. Because it is low impact, you can do it virtually every day and not stress your body.

Running or Jogging

Running or jogging.

What's the difference?

Speed. I think runners run at a pace of eight minutes per mile or less. Many runners run at a six-minute-mile pace.

Joggers are slower, usually running at a pace of eight to ten minutes per mile.

You only need to be a jogger to be successful with running as a Thirty-Minute Fitness activity.

Get a good pair of running shoes and some foul-weather gear, and you are set.

The key to running or jogging with Thirty-Minute Fitness is to begin your run immediately when you step out your front door.

Don't drive down to the park or local scenic jogging area. Why? That adds too much time.

Just go out your front door, and run or jog for twenty to twenty-two minutes.

That's it.

Other Activities

So I've discussed my holy trinity of aerobic exercises—swimming, walking, and biking.

Running or jogging is the fourth exercise in the big four of the aerobic exercise world.

The most important reason that I have picked these exercises is not necessarily because they are the best.

It's because they are generally the easiest and most efficient exercises to do. That is, they are relatively frictionless.

By frictionless, I mean you can start them immediately and not waste a lot of time transitioning from one activity to another, getting equipment on, or going to a different location to do it.

Now, swimming in a pool does require you to go to a pool, but because it's such a great aerobic exercise, I find the transportation time worthwhile.

You get great results from these four basic activities. **But don't let my favorite big four activities limit you.**

You may want to add to the list: working out on an elliptical machine, going cross-country skiing in the winter, or doing some form of circuit training. They're all just as good and equally simple to do.

There is a world of other aerobic activities to do. Handball, racquetball, basketball, volleyball, tennis, stair running, Zumba, dancing, and circuit training come to mind. They all qualify.

Craft your own holy trinity of exercise routines that you can use in your Thirty Minute Fitness program on a regular basis. And then start doing them.

Remember, they need to be enjoyable for you to do and also be activities that you can do quickly and without a lot of preparation or wasted time.

OTHER ISSUES

Eat Half

Many Americans are overweight.

We eat and eat and eat. We eat long after the point of fullness or satiety where we have eaten enough for our body's nutritional needs.

Many Americans are also on diets. Diets work sometimes, and sometimes they don't.

If you put a TMF exercise program in place, you also need to curb your appetite. Or at least put a circuit breaker in place to help you not eat too much.

This isn't a diet book. It's an exercise book. So there's nothing here about dieting, how to diet, and what you should diet with. Diet books run into the thousands, and there are both good and bad diets out there.

There is a much simpler approach to food control in two words: eat half.

Eat half. Either do it literally and lose a ton of weight quickly, or do it as a mind-set. Many people use this approach and only eat half of the food on their plate consistently. They know, rightly so, that we Americans eat vast quantities of food—primarily junk food and carbohydrates—that can be downsized immediately and we would still function perfectly. It works fabulously for many people, and it's an approach that may work for you, too.

I could never do that, cold turkey. It's almost impossible to just eat half when you start. I would be ravenous by two in the afternoon if I ate only 50 percent of my lunch.

But I do eat less on my plate consistently and do it fairly easily. When you're at a business lunch, and they have those half-cut sandwiches, only take one. It works. Also leave some chips in the bag and then eat only half of a cookie. Give the other half to a colleague.

Some people always end their meal by leaving a little food on their plate. It forces them to eat 10 to 15 percent less. They train themselves, and it works. Whenever I leave a small amount of food on my plate, I still feel satisfied and full at the end of the meal. This practice makes you realize that you probably put too much food on your plate in the first place.

You may also find that pausing after a salad or an appetizer, sometimes even pausing during the meal, works very effectively at appetite control.

Also try eating a little slower. It gives your brain time to catch up with your stomach to tell it that it's

had enough. Otherwise, you can eat and eat and eat. Trust me on this!

And it's that marginal eating that puts all the weight on, before your brain tells your stomach that it's full and no more food is needed.

So just eat half as a lifestyle. Walk away from the rest.

Mediterranean Diet

Nothing is perfect out there.

This is particularly true when it comes to food, diets, and all the things that you should be eating and that are healthy for you.

That said, the Mediterranean diet is rising up through many medical and dietary journals as being a great protocol for protecting you from long-term physical issues including heart attack, stroke, and high blood pressure.

That all sounds too good to be true. But as I finish this book in the fall of 2013, a major new study on the Mediterranean diet has just come out. The scientists running the study concluded it early, because the diet was shown to be so conclusively beneficial to long-term health that the testing did not need to be prolonged. So there it is.

What is the Mediterranean diet? It's a combination of things. It's eating a handful of mixed nuts every day. Having olive oil with your meal and eating lots of green vegetables, legumes, and fruit. Meat

is generally used as an additive to meals, rather than the meal itself.

All these items are generally common sense and not difficult at all to incorporate into your diet.

You also need to try to get rid of all processed foods, which continue to hold sway over most of us.

So the Mediterranean diet may be something that you want to incorporate into your Thirty-Minute Fitness campaign.

Alcohol

There is nothing wrong with having a beer or a glass of wine or whatever kind of drink you enjoy.

I enjoy alcohol and try to use it moderately. Alcohol, when used moderately, can have a positive effect on your health.

Again, moderation is the key.

Drinking red wine, for example, in moderation has been proved to be beneficial to your long-term health. How much is moderate? Probably about one generous glass, which is about seven to eight ounces of liquid. One cup is six ounces, so use a measuring cup to measure a cupful and a little more.

I also think that drinking a beer with a meal is a lot better than drinking a soda, which contains about twelve teaspoons of sugar in each twelve-ounce can. But drinking alcohol during the business day is generally frowned upon.

So you won't find a screed against alcohol in Thirty-Minute Fitness. However, there are a lot of carbohydrates in alcohol. If you are a beer drinker, you can put weight on fairly easily.

So enjoy alcohol in a responsible way. But realize that less is probably more, particularly if you are exercising with a Thirty-Minute Fitness routine four or five times a week.

Salt and Sugar

What needs to be said about these two highly addictive substances?

As Americans, we ingest voracious amounts of sugar and salt. An article in the *New York Times* recently said that Americans consume about twenty-two teaspoons of sugar a day. A day! Think about that for a minute.

The same is true for salt. We eat more than twice the daily recommended amount of sodium in our diets.

But it is not all our fault.

Food scientists have become wizards at lacing bad food with sugar and salt additives and other chemicals to make it taste incredibly good. Too good, in fact, for us to stop eating it—particularly when we should have stopped long ago.

I think sugar and salt are as addictive as alcohol and have devastating effects on our bodies over the long term. But for some strange reason, being an alcoholic is shunned in our society, but being addicted to sugar or salt is treated benignly. Our kids are particularly susceptible to sugar and salt addictions at an early age.

I am addicted to sugar and salt, myself. I try to cut back, but it's difficult. Cheez-Its, Oreos, Doritos, and potato chips are among my worst eating habits.

If you are doing Thirty-Minute Fitness regularly, try to cut down on sugar and salt in your diet. This can eliminate the blood-sugar spikes that often go along with eating all this junk.

And since all the foods we eat are loaded with salt and sugar straight from the package, we never need to add those to our diet.

If you are successful in just cutting down a little on salt and sugar in your diet, the rewards will be plentiful.

To start, you will feel much better.

And just as important, you will have much more energy for your Thirty-Minute Fitness program, which will make it that much easier to maintain your exercise routine.

Sleep

Can you ever get too much sleep when you are exercising? Probably not.

Be sure to maintain an adequate sleep schedule when you are doing Thirty-Minute Fitness.

It is not just important. It's critical.

Many of us exist on six hours of sleep a night. I sometimes sleep even less, getting by on about

five and a half hours a night. But I nap on weekends if I can, to try to replenish. It never works.

We Americans are generally sleep deprived and stressed by the twin pillars of family and jobs. Existing on less sleep is seen as a good thing, a positive skill.

It is not. Most of us are in a perpetual state of severe sleep deprivation.

If you are doing Thirty-Minute Fitness regularly, the program will drain the energy from your tank if you are not sleeping enough. While thirty minutes is a small amount of time to spend exercising and the routine is not too taxing, its repetitiveness uses a lot of energy.

Sleep is the only way to replenish that energy. So try to get seven to eight hours of sleep a night if you are serious about doing Thirty-Minute Fitness. You will need it.

Now, here's the good part. Are you an insomniac and have trouble sleeping at night? A lot of people are.

Thirty-Minute Fitness may help you to sleep more each night. Why? Because you'll frequently be tired.

Regular exercise uses a lot of energy. TMF may force you into a more beneficial sleep cycle as your body will need the replenishment of sleep along the way.

WRAP-UP

Thirty-Minute Fitness Redux

Simplicity and regularity.

That is the essence of the Thirty-Minute Fitness program.

TMF is, at its core, simple.

There are no DVDs to put into your DVD player or laptop to watch, because who has the time to watch DVDs?

There isn't any bulky equipment to buy. No iPad or iPhone applications to tap with exercises loaded in.

No special routines or programs to memorize and repeat.

Just get out there four or five days a week and do ten minutes of light exercise or weight training and then do twenty minutes of aerobic activity like running or walking or biking.

That's it!

It sounds simple and simplistic—probably because it is.

The benefits you will gain in terms of fitness attained will be amazing.

You will feel better than you have in years. You will become active and in shape. This will happen quickly, as in the first thirty to forty-five days.

Keep it up, and you will have created a platform on which to live for years in good health going forward.

Remember the TMF Routine

Remember the elements of Thirty-Minute Fitness.

Each one is important to your overall fitness goals. They are all interlocking. When taken together, they are the secret sauce that will allow you to exercise successfully over the short and the long term.

The keys are:

- There are two parts to the routine: first part work and then aerobic activity.
- Exercise for no more than thirty minutes a day. If you do too much, you will most likely quit at some point. Do not quit. Thirty minutes is a great psychological touchstone. It is an endpoint, a reference point. Everyone can exercise for thirty minutes.
- On some days, do six to ten minutes of exercising, including core work and basic calisthenics to start. This means doing things like jumping jacks, half push-ups, and leg lifts. Keep them light and easy.

Do sets of five to ten repetitions per exercise to keep your form excellent and precise.

- On other days, do six to ten minutes of weight training. Include things like side raises, military presses, bench presses, and behind-the-head pullovers. Use light dumbbells of ten pounds each and keep your form excellent and precise. Do sets of five to seven repetitions per exercise.

- Then do twenty minutes of aerobic work. Keep it simple and do something like a walk, jog, run, or bike. Possibly include swimming or some other complementary activity. Be able to walk out your door and begin this part of your exercising with little or no transition or downtime so that you don't waste any time.

- Do your Thirty-Minute Fitness routine four or five times a week consistently. Make it part of your daily routine.

- Do not quit. Ever.

- Enjoy your workout by doing exercises, weight training, and aerobic activities that you personally like to do. Nothing should be drudgery.

- Constantly mix up your routine and cross-train. Don't do the same thing repetitively. Change it up!

-

That's it. Do the Thirty-Minute Fitness routine for the rest of your life, and you will stay in shape with a minimum amount of energy spent and will likely enjoy good health along the way.

What else can you ask for in life?

Never Give Up

I put this chapter here, near the end, because it's probably the most important exercise tip in the book. It's critical, not just important.

Persevere. Never give up on your Thirty-Minute Fitness plan.

This is the psychological cornerstone in your TMF program going forward. Everything builds off of it.

One of the key elements in Thirty-Minute Fitness is its maximum time for exercise—thirty minutes.

Why? Because you run the risk of quitting your exercise routine if it's longer. If you exercise for forty-five minutes to an hour, you are a lot more likely to quit your routine if something happens. Or do less exercising.

And remember, something will always happen in your life. Your job will require you to spend more time in the office. Your significant other or spouse or kids will take more of your time. Housework, errands, laundry, and the dog will compromise your ability to exercise regularly.

Never stop and never give up in spite of these obstacles.

Your Thirty-Minute Fitness routine should be a nonnegotiable part of your life from now on. Why? Because it's only thirty minutes!

Everybody has thirty minutes to devote to a fitness plan four or five times a week. Everybody. It needs to be a priority for you, on an equal footing with your job and family and friends.

Never give up. Never stop.

Only by making Thirty-Minute Fitness an essential part of your daily life will you become fit and stay in shape for the long term.

Enjoy!

Lastly, your workouts should be a pleasure in your daily routine—a small joy. You should look forward to them. They should dissipate the stress in your life.

You've got to enjoy doing your Thirty-Minute Fitness routine every day.

How do you do that? It's easy!

Only do exercises and activities that you like, that are simple, and that are easy and efficient to do.

If you don't like lifting weights, then don't do that activity much.

Hate exercises and calisthenics?

Only do a select few that you really need to stay in shape (like working on your core), and instead spend more of your time doing light weight lifting.

Don't like running? Then walk.

Don't like swimming? Never swim.

It's simple—you've got to enjoy whatever it is you do for exercise in your TMF routine.

And by enjoying your routine and keeping it short (thirty minutes or less!), you will be more likely to do it regularly and be successful.

Results

You will definitely see and feel results quickly with this program.

Guaranteed.

Will you lose twenty pounds and drop two inches in your waist?

That's not likely unless you adjust your eating habits and caloric consumption significantly.

Can you lose two inches off your waist with Thirty Minute Fitness? Possibly. But losing two inches is not what this program is all about. If that is really your goal, you should be on a different kind of exercise and weight loss plan.

But…

- **If you measure results in terms of having energy to burn during your workday and then at home, TMF is your solution.**
- **If feeling fit and being in shape is your goal, TMF will help.**

- **If getting basic muscle tone and flexibility is important, TMF is your roadmap to success.**

Lifting weights the Thirty Minute Fitness way will help you tighten and tone your upper body, arms, and shoulders.

And the walking and running component will give your legs basic definition and strength.

All the various activities that you do here as part of your Thirty-Minute Fitness routine will act in tandem to bring you overall good health and body fitness. You will get toned and tight as you exercise frequently, but for shorter periods.

You will not get bulky or muscular—just toned and tight. And that is just the way you want to be.

Cross-training and varying your routine will also help. Cross-training is a key antidote for boredom and will keep your workouts interesting and fun.

The Beginning

So there you have it: a lifetime exercise and fitness plan in under one hundred and fifty pages.

Exercise isn't rocket science.

But it takes a strong and disciplined mind to do it regularly and effectively.

The Thirty-Minute Fitness plan is a program that will lead to fundamental fitness and will help you get and stay in shape. But you've got to follow the routine and do it frequently.

So this is the beginning, not the end.

It is the beginning of your Thirty-Minute Fitness plan, which you will craft for yourself to get fit and stay in shape—for the long haul.

Do the routine. Enjoy the activity.

The key to success is to start doing the TMF routine today. Not tomorrow. Today.

Try it out and see if it doesn't make a minor, or possibly major, difference in your life.

Start today to get in shape the Thirty-Minute Fitness way. Good luck.

John Moynihan
Brookline Village, Ma.
January 2014

Made in the USA
Charleston, SC
13 January 2014